Yoga for beginners
99 Reasons to do Yoga?

Personal Development for women

by

Sammy Hermans

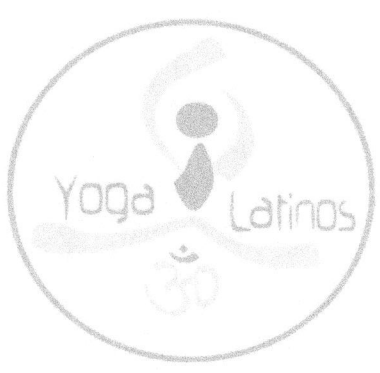

Copyright

You agree to accept all risks of using the information in this book. You are advised to consult a professional medical practitioner in order to ensure you are able and healthy enough to participate in this program.

The reader should regularly consult a physician in matters relating to his or her health.

Contents

How will this book benefit YOU?

You will:

- Understand why you have to start with Yoga Today,
- Learn how Yoga will benefit your health,
- Find out how Yoga will give you more flexibility,
- Get encouraged to change your life in a positive way,
- Feel better after reading this book,
- Start learning what to do to enjoy life,
- Know what road to take to become happier,
- Have more confidence when you finished this book to start with Yoga,
- Make a switch to your lifestyle in a positive direction,
- Accomplish a new way of thinking,
- Motivate yourself to become a better person,
- Have fun by reading this easy to read book,
- Understand why Yoga can change your life Today in the healthy way.

Thank You

I would like to begin this book by thanking you to read one of the books I have written to change your life. I know your time is valuable and I am very grateful that you decided to take a little time out of your day to read my book. I am sure you will be happy after reading this 99 reasons to start with Yoga.

Thank You and enjoy!

The author

Sammy Hermans is an upcoming author that was born in the early 80's and has since childhood a great interest in the Yoga art. He was studying multiple Yoga styles and grew up in Belgium, the capital of Europe. The author is a real world citizen and likes to get new influences from all over the world.

The author loves to do research about the different Yoga styles to implement them in the Yoga classes and help people to find the best Yoga styles that fits them.

Meditation has helped him gain control over his mind and live a stress-free, more productive, healthy and happier life. Sammy enjoys seeing the wonderful improvements in peoples lives through Yoga.

He loves to help people with this new lifestyle and guide them through this healthy journey. The author is always willing to help people to become happier and healthier.

The author started a Yoga training and Yoga coaching business together with his partner Sherley Henry De Hermans. The company 'Yoga Latinos' was created to help people along their journey towards a healthy Yoga life.

Together they are willing to help and guide everybody in their new mindset. Please checkout www.yogalatinos.com if you are interested in more Yoga information on the blog or if you are interested in online Yoga classes.

Sammy's other interests include world music, dancing, relaxing and meditation, multimedia arts, reading, traveling, spending time in nature & drinking cups of tea and enjoying time with his wife, kids and family.

Discover all the amazing ideas in his books.

References

The information in this book was created thanks to the knowledge gained through the years of studying and practicing the Yoga art.

Some of the information and guidelines are created with the knowledge conserved and gained by reading following books:

- *V. Worthington, A History of Yoga, Arkana, London,1982,*

- *S.Swami, Asana Pranayama Mudra Bandha, Yoga Publications Trust,India 2002,*

- *Surendranath, D., A History of Indian Philosophy, Cambridge University Press, 1955,*

- *G. Feuerstein, The Yoga Tradition, Hohm Press, Arizona, 2001.*

The true method of knowledge is experiment.

Thanks and Credits

Thanks to everybody that supported me with writing this Yoga book. Special thanks goes to my partner Sherley Henry De Hermans. She helped with research and advice to accomplish the 99 reasons to do Yoga

Sherley Henry De Hermans is a Yoga teacher for the company Yoga Latinos and has several years of experience with teaching different Yoga styles and knows different poses and techniques. However she mainly concentrates on Hatha Yoga, Vinyasa Yoga, Ashantha Yoga and Dance Yoga, but she is also an expert in massage and pressure point techniques.

If you are looking for professional help and a perfect guide during your Yoga journey, you can contact Sherley on www.yogalatinos.com for online Yoga classes.

Together we are a Yoga team and we are willing to help you with all your health problems or just getting you to the next Yoga level.

The attitude of gratitude is the highest Yoga.

A helping hand for the author

Thank you for purchasing this book and reading it. I hope you will be happy with the "99 reasons to do Yoga" book. You are now ready to start your journey throughout the Yoga world.

In order to make it possible to do more research and to write more books, it is important to get your full support. You can help a lot by putting some honest reviews on the website www.yogalatinos.com or on the Amazon Kindle book reviews.

Please keep in mind that by giving a honest five star rate, you will support the author. If you like the book "99 Reasons to do Yoga", and you want to read more Yoga related books, please check out the other books written by the same author, Sammy Hermans, such as "How to lose 10 pounds in 10 days with Yoga?" got to the Amazon webshop.

Some other titles you will like, are: "How to control your kids with Yoga?", "The Yoga body book", "Happy Yoga", "Loving pregnancy thanks to Yoga" and more coming.

Every time that you buy a book from the author, you are supporting the author to do more research and write more books that can help you in different ways.

Every book can give you more insights to Yoga and can help you for a more healthy and happier life. If you have any suggestions or comments, you can report them any time by filling in the contact form at the website www.yogalatinos.com. Please support.

Thanks a lot for the support!

Prologue: Why Yoga?

'Yoga', the term derived from the Sanskrit word 'Yuj', which means 'to unite' or 'to join'. It is an art, a system which signifies the unification or integration of body, soul and mind in harmony.

The meaning of this word itself is the epitome of its power and benefits that it provides to its disciples. Yogis in gradual practice discover various benefits of Yoga and a sincere practitioner tends to achieve the highest of them.

Today this practice is no niche, in fact it is currently enveloping the whole world under its cover. People have begun to realize its importance and intellectuals.

Yogis, and different Global health organizations are enforcing the reasons to start practicing Yoga. With media and internet at their rage, nobody can stay aloof of this beautiful concept.

However, here in this small ebook you will find the most prominent 99 reasons to do Yoga, that will definitely encourage you to adopt this practice. You can read other books written by the same author, these books will dive deeper in some specific benefits.

Find out Your 99 Reasons to do Yoga

The 99 Reasons to do Yoga

1) Yoga has numerous exercises and poses which strengthens our muscles.

2) Yoga helps in toning of the muscles.

3) Yoga improves our respiration system through its various exercises focusing on breathing; especially, meditation.

4) Yoga exercises are such that they will make your entire body flexible and agile.

5) It has been proved that Yoga has really magical effects on curing different body pains such as back ache, headache, knee pain and so on.

6) Yoga is unusually known to be a supportive therapy in treatment of some grievous and fatal diseases like Cancer by reducing the patient's pain, increasing will power and positivism.

7) Yoga is known to cure various diseases which are nowadays very common like heart diseases, asthma, arthritis, cough and cold and many more.

8) Its regular practice increases our immune power tremendously and we tend to fall less sick even to the seasonal diseases like flu, viral fever, and so on.

9) Yoga revitalizes you and help in regaining the energy whenever you feel tired and exhausted.

10) Yoga is a great stress reliever since its practice helps in release of the positive chemical called endorphin which boosts our mood and helps us in overcoming stress levels.

11) It is a great way to come out from the dark phase of depression since it helps in pulling out the negative emotions and inducing the positive ones in the mind.

12) Yoga is known to help people in reducing the anxiety levels to a great extent.

13) One of the most significant reason of practicing Yoga is that, it makes your attitude positive and helps you to focus only on the positives of the situation.

14) Yoga is a great teacher of Mind-Control. It teaches how to control our thoughts and emotions.

15) Because of Yoga we learn to stay and live in the present. This enables us to dwell less on the past and not to worry about the future.

16) Yoga practice helps in increasing the self-confidence which is very necessary to attain success, be it professionally or socially.

17) Yoga is said to increase our self-esteem as well. It is one such practice which teaches us to accept ourselves as we are and respect our own selves.

18) Yoga not only increases the self-esteem but helps in encouraging oneself to further improve in life.

19) Yoga also helps in increasing self-awareness to the highest levels which helps us in determining our strengths and weaknesses.

20) Yoga also increases one's alertness and consciousness to the outer world.

21) Yoga helps bringing discipline into one's life.

22) Yoga is thus also a very great way of knowing what is right and what is morally wrong.

23) Yoga is based on the principle of 'Ahimsa' or 'Nonviolence' which teaches us not to cause harm to any living beings, even the animals.

24) Yoga teaches us to follow rules in order to balance the nature.

25) Yoga teaches us to respect our mother nature and changes our outlook towards it by encouraging us to restrict the use of resources and return to it as well.

26) The concepts of self-awareness and consciousness of outer world enables us to become more compassionate and to think about returning to the society and work for its benefits.

27) Yoga helps in developing relationship of love and understanding between us and our body.

28) It also helps in listening to our own body calls and work towards them.

29) Yoga helps in throwing away the burden of all the guilt and traumas of the past. Thus making us happier.

30) It helps in fighting from negative emotions like anger, envy, jealousy and frustration through its exercises and the magical practice of meditation.

31) Yoga brings internal peace and calmness in the body.

32) Yoga helps in a great way to cure insomnia and increases the quality of sleep.

33) One more good reason for practicing Yoga is when you really want to stop those heavy dosage of medications like antidepressants, steroids and so on and be healthier naturally.

34) It also teaches the Yogic principle of 'Karma' which helps in performing good and kind deeds.

35) Yoga although is a free system and doesn't enforce anything on you, but it is based on principles like 'Ahimsa' and 'Karma' and eating those foods which does not cause any harm to the body, promotes the consumption of 'Sattvic' diet i.e. Vegetarian diet.

36) Consumption of meat is quite a harmful diet as it is one of the greatest source of cholesterol, a heart killer, and also is very difficult to digest. So Yoga promoting a vegetarian diet really helps the Yogi staying healthier.

37) Yoga helps in increasing the life expectancy.

38) Yoga helps in controlling the blood pressure.

39) Yoga also improves the blood circulation thus keeping us energetic and healthy.

40) Yoga practice is known to be significantly improving the nervous system of the body.

41) We in our lives tend to consume many things that increases the toxic levels of our body. Yoga as a practice and the diet that it recommends really helps in detoxification of the body.

42) It is a great way to learn to balance. Practicing different Yoga poses like tree pose, Child pose and so on really improves the balance of the body.

43) Yoga is also known for improving the coordination skills through its various exercises and poses.

44) Yoga improves our posture.

45) Also, Yoga is really very beneficial for the kids. It improves their motor skills and concentration levels.

46) Yoga practice among kids helps in enhancing their brain power greatly and increases the mental ability's development rate.

47) Yoga is a great way to fight obesity. It helps tremendously in reducing the weight.

48) It also improves our digestion system which is the main cause of many diseases and discomforts caused to the body.

49) Yoga helps in maintaining and balancing our body metabolism.

50) Yoga has some great exercises for eyes too, a very important part of our body and senses. It relaxes them and increases their strength.

51) Yoga is a great way to reduce the sodium which enters our body through the junk and adulterated food consumption.

52) Amazingly, regular practice of Yoga is said to increase the Red Blood Cells in our body. Thus, it prevents from being anemic.

53) Also, if we go deeper into the biochemistry kind of benefits of Yoga than it its regular practice also helps in reduction of triglycerides which are form of fat and are harmful for our heart's functioning.

54) Yoga regimen is also said to maintain and balance the hormone's secretion in proper levels in the body thus making you healthier.

55) Yoga also improves the memory as it regulates the blood supply to the brain as well.

56) It burns fat and lowers down the cholesterol levels.

57) Studies also show that Yoga exercises and meditation together are very effective in improving the reaction time of the body.

58) Sportsmen and athletes are highly recommended to practice Yoga since it significantly improves the endurance levels.

59) A special mention to the disease of Alzheimer, which is really a worst of the diseases a human suffers from. Yoga is said to enhance the brain gamma-amino butyric (GABA) levels which are very helpful for the cure of the disease.

60) Yoga also helps in curing of diabetes by maintaining the glucose levels in the body.

61) With increasing pollution and adulteration in food as well, there are increasing numbers of people falling prone to allergies. Yoga helps magically in eliminating these allergic symptoms.

62) Even the deadly disease of Epileptic Seizures is known to get prevented by the regular Yoga practice.

63) Yoga is very helpful for women especially since it affects greatly in reducing the side effects of menopause.

64) Not only menopause but it is very helpful for relieving from the discomforts during the menstruation period.

65) Migraines has to have a special mention since they are found to be very irritating form of pain. Yoga greatly helps in their prevention and cure as well. Meditation too works wonders here.

66) We all worry about aging effects, and following a regular Yoga regimen will reduce this effects and delay the aging process.

67) It improves our sexual functions as well.

68) Yoga also helps us in becoming successful socially as it leads not only our inner awareness but our awareness to the society as well.

69) It improves your intuition power.

70) Regular practice of Yoga leads you to deeper realization and thus improves your wisdom as well.

71) Yoga has some very good exercises for hair health as well.

72) Yoga can make your skin glow naturally and become more beautiful.

73) It helps in boosting up our mood while in crisis situation by a simple practice of mediation for few minutes.

74) Yoga is a system which teaches us to become more organized in our life.

75) Yoga is also known for healing injuries more smoothly and faster.

76) Yoga not only works up on muscles but also on soft tissues like tendons and ligaments and keeps them well maintained.

77) Yoga increases not only our physical stamina but also our mental stamina.

78) Yoga also helps in maintaining a healthy spine curvature.

79) Yoga actually increases our core strength.

80) Although yoga induces discipline in our lives but it also empowers us to explore more of our lives thus making us sense complete freedom and delight.

81) Yoga is also claimed that it really supports the recovery of stroke and paralytic patients.

82) Regular practice of Yoga even empowers us to venture out from our comfort zone and be comfortable even in odd situations.

83) Yoga greatly helps in reducing panic attacks.

84) Yoga is really helpful to rise emotionally from negative phases and grief of our lives such as losing someone to death or broken relationships and so on.

85) Yoga also helps in forming and maintaining a healthy relationship with others.

86) Practice of Yoga will make you always feel lighter.

87) Yoga greatly helps us in overcoming the laziness and sluggishness.

88) Yoga is a very proven way whose practice really makes one embrace the changes and challenges in life more easily.

89) It is said that the Yoga is a spiritual experience and thus brings enlightenment and bliss with itself.

90) And practicing Yoga itself means that you are devoting time for your own selves and it is really a great way of expressing gratitude towards our body.

91) Yoga helps greatly in clearing one's self-doubts.

92) It is also said that a regular practitioner of Yoga attains a gracefulness and poise which makes him or her a very attractive personality as well.

93) Yoga is known to relieve discomfort during the pregnancy of the women.

94) It is also said to be greatly effective in painless and smooth delivery and even after delivery stages discomforts.

95) Yoga is easily accessible. You can learn it sitting at your home by watching Yoga Tutorials or join a Yoga group or a Yoga class.

96) Yoga can be practiced almost anywhere, indoors as well as outdoors. Some exercises can even be done while sitting at your workplace desk.

97) Yoga helps in changing your perspectives and attitude towards life in a very positive way.

98) Yoga induces greater tolerance and stability in our behavior.

99) And most importantly Yoga shows how to live the life to the fullest and in a happier way.

So, how many more reasons do one want to start practicing Yoga right off? There are many reasons that would have instantly got connected to you and your experiences and would really encourage you to adopt this regimen.

Ultimately it is going to be a really beneficial routine for you. So go, get yourself buckled up, for experiencing a wonderful life with the practice of the magical 'Yoga'!

Start Your Yoga Life Today!

Check out this amazing book

Tired from all the diet programs that promise you to lose weight fast? Do you need a real solution for your weight problems? Buy Now on Amazon this amazing book about weight loss, "How to lose 10 pounds in 10 days with Yoga?" on the Amazon webshop.

By reading this book you will:

- Lose fat fast
- Get Stress Relief
- Show your friends and family the positive changes from this Yoga Diet
- Stay in a healthy shape
- Make positive changes to your physical and mental health
- Start an amazing new lifestyle
- Become more aware of yourself

Start Now and do what all healthy Celebrities are doing! Put on your Yoga pants to start losing weight Today. "How to lose 10 pounds in 10 DAYS with Yoga?" will open up a new world for You.

Get started with the basic principles from the Yoga art. You will feel the difference from the first day with this Yoga plan for beginners.

You will feel better in many ways thanks to Yoga for beginners. Be ready for the positive influence that Yoga will bring into Your life. Get ready and change things starting from Today!

Now is the time to start losing weight fast. It will not be suffering like how so many other programs let you do, it will be easy to lose weight fast!

Yoga is easy and will change you with little efforts. I promise you that the Yoga lifestyle will make a big difference in your life. People will ask you what is it that made you change?

You will be able to show your weight loss to friends and let them join the Yoga diet program and have more fun. Because this 10 days program can be done over and over, you will easily continue with following your new lifestyle with this Yoga for beginners program.

Get your mind ready and your body will follow.Don't worry, you can do this, everybody can. Yoga is not only for flexible people, it will make you flexible. Yoga is not for the physically strong, it will make you stronger along the way.

Get started today with losing weight. Don't hesitate to get started, every day you wait is a day lost. I'm sure you will regret you didn't start earlier with this Yoga weight loss program. YES you are ready for this!

This book is a:

- Step by step program that makes you feel better
- Guide to start losing weight from the first day
- Perfect way to start with meditation and mindfulness

Put on some Yoga clothing or sport clothes or just work out in something comfortable. Get your Yoga mat or just practice on a solid non slippery floor.

If you think you don't have the space to do yoga at home or there is always too much noise, you can just go outside and practice in a park, forest or on the beach.

Start the 10 days program and you will lose fat fast before you know it with this Yoga Diet. You will be so happy and satisfied with this fantastic way of losing weight. You will be surprised what this Yoga book can do for you, your friends and family. Try it out Now and Enjoy! Order now on the Amazon webshop.

Please don't force yourself, but start open minded.

Extra Bonus

Because I am so happy that you were reading all of my book, I will give you the first chapter from my book "How to lose 10 pounds in 10 days with Yoga?" completely for Free so you can enjoy it already. If you want to buy it check it out in the Amazon webshop.

Chapter 1 from the book "How to lose 10 pounds in 10 days with Yoga?": Can the 10 DAYS program really work for me?

Many people believe that weight loss arises from excessively strict dieting, strenuous cardio and even weight training; Yoga may frequently be overlooked as an option for weight loss as it is not commonly thought of as a slimming exercise.

However, Yoga should be considered for weight loss as there are many benefits to participating in this exercise. Yoga allows for participants to strengthen their inner core muscles and build strength.

Whilst this form of exercise may not burn an extensive amount of calories, it allows for the individual to train their mind to make healthier choices.

This new way of healthier thinking promotes healthy choices relating to the individual's body, such as the decision to eat healthier foods and participate in more regular physical activity.

Whilst Yoga traditionally does not burn the calories that walking or running does, Yoga helps a person increase their own mindfulness, particularly how they think of and relate to their own self and body.

For example, regular participation in Yoga allows one to develop a deep sense of understanding about their body, and even a connection with themselves and their health. An avid Yoga participant will be aware of how they are feeling internally, and additionally will understand what foods make their body feel better or worse.

This will help to promote healthier choices in relation to the consumption of certain foods; therefore, Yoga, through promoting an awareness of yourself, promotes healthy eating choices and therefore weight loss.

A common question posed by many who are unfamiliar with Yoga and the related benefits is often "can Yoga really work for me?" The answer is simple: **YES!**

Yoga can work for anyone who is open to participating in an activity that will allow the person to relate to and connect with their body. "Can this 10 days Yoga food and Yoga exercise program work for me?" The answer is **YES!**

Here's why: Primarily, Yoga involves continuous use of your muscles, which burns calories. This means that your muscles are continuously stretching and working, which means you are exercising, which in turn promotes weight loss.

So, as a result, this aspect of participating in the activity alone means Yoga will work for you as a form of weight loss!

Furthermore, this program only requires 15 minutes of Yoga exercise a day, so it's easy to participate and get motivated!The second aspect of this 10 days program is the food. Following this diet that has been provided to you will not only decrease your calorie intake to a healthier level, but will also promote an increase in your metabolism, thus enhancing weight loss.

Weight loss typically occurs when a person's calorie intake is less than their calorie expenditure. Simply put, if you burn more calories than you eat, your body will be forced to burn its own fat storage, causing you to lose weight.

The foods chosen in this 10 days Yoga food and Yoga exercise program are designed to work in combination with a Yoga exercise program to maximize your weight loss! The particular foods have been proven to satisfy hunger and cravings even though they are low in calories; the perfect combination for weight loss!

The food chosen for this Yoga food and Yoga exercise program are portioned in realistic sizes, unlike many other diets that leave you feeling hungry. After reading the book you should be able to learn more about your own body and feel when to stop eating; in order to avoid eating too many calories.

This program considers the individual; foods have been chosen that are tasty and won't make you feel like you're on a 10 days diet. Most people may even continue the food plan after the 10 days because it is a realistic way that is not a diet, but a lifestyle and a way of eating healthier. The results speak for themselves and you will see these results yourself after your 10 days participation!

In conclusion, will this program work for you? The answer is, **Yes.** This 10 days Yoga food and Yoga exercise program will have you connect with your inner self and make healthier choices that promote weight loss. This program will promote daily exercise to tone and tighten your body in combination with a diet that will speed up your metabolism and burn fat.

The program will work for you because even from day 1 you will feel as though you are not on a diet or completing a rigorous exercise scheme, but rather you are making a life change to improve your overall health and well being; what could possible feel better than that?

Change Your Life Now Thanks to Yoga!

Book tags

yoga, yoga for beginners, yoga diet, stress relief, meditation, beginners, inner peace, mindfulness, Yoga, anxiety, mood management, restore the balance, weight loss guide, stress, books, mindfulness meditation, yoga guide, meditation for beginners, meditation books, yoga books, zen meditation, how to meditate, ashtanga yoga, hatha yoga, vinyasa yoga, self-help, increase productivity, daily meditations, yoga for weight loss, relieve stress, yoga anatomy, spiritual growth, yoga stress relief, yoga, yoga for beginners, yoga for meditation, helpful books, books for life, health books, diet, asana, ashtanga, bhakti, Buddha, drishti, guru, karma, karuna, kula, prana, agami karma, sun salutation, standing poses, balancing poses, sitting poses, halasana, salamba sarvangasana, tadasana, utkatasana, ustrasana, savasana, boat pose, bow pose, bridge pose, basic poses, utkatasana, modified downward facing dog, warrior pose, half moon pose, sun, motivation, groving, weight loss every day, training program, diet books, healthy living, outdoor, yoga at home, meditation for stress relief, tired, yoga for women, advanced Yoga, energy, active, yoga for beginners, healthy food, detox, diet plan, organic food, overweight, feel better, motivate yourself, diet program that helps, yoga books for beginners, yoga, weight loss book, losing weight thanks to yoga, meditation outside, happy, family, teaching, coaching, relax, relaxation, kids yoga, yoga for women above 50, yoga for advanced, yogi, better life, younger, health benefits, improve, more, no more damage, food choices, veggie, vegetarian, diet for weight loss, yoga world, yoga classes, yoga for pregnant women, yoga for baby's, yoga all day, thanks, mudras, mudras for beginners, chakras, chakras for advanced, meditation for beginners, mind, body, soul, spirit, light, heart, feelings, good, great, yoga love, healthy mind, mind-control, yoga breathing, breath controlling, becoming young again, youth, yoga spirit, yoga journey, music, yoga music, yoga mood, yoga meditations, yoga for yogi, food that is good, happy food, yoga happy food, important, self-awareness, self-doubts, relationship, practicing yoga, panic attacks, discipline, strenght, increase health, deeper wisdom, burn fat fast, burn belly fat, yoga diet book, yoga health program, yoga results, yoga beginner, improve memory, memory training, brain power, blood pressure, cardio, alertness, yoga forever, yoga symbols, cure, yoga basic poses, yoga in the morning, yoga breakfast, yoga cadio, yoga for weight loss book, yoga diet program, yoga, diet food, energy food, growing up with yoga, yoga for weight problems, feel good yoga, yoga mental power, yoga inner peace, yoga body, yoga cures, yoga systems for weight loss, lose weight fast, yoga energy, yoga breath control, yoga course, yoga peace, yoga program for health problems,yoga, yogi